AMERICA'S RECIPES
——HUB——

THE MOST DELICIOUS

KALORIK

MAXX

RECIPES

Collection

Every day easy Fish recipes

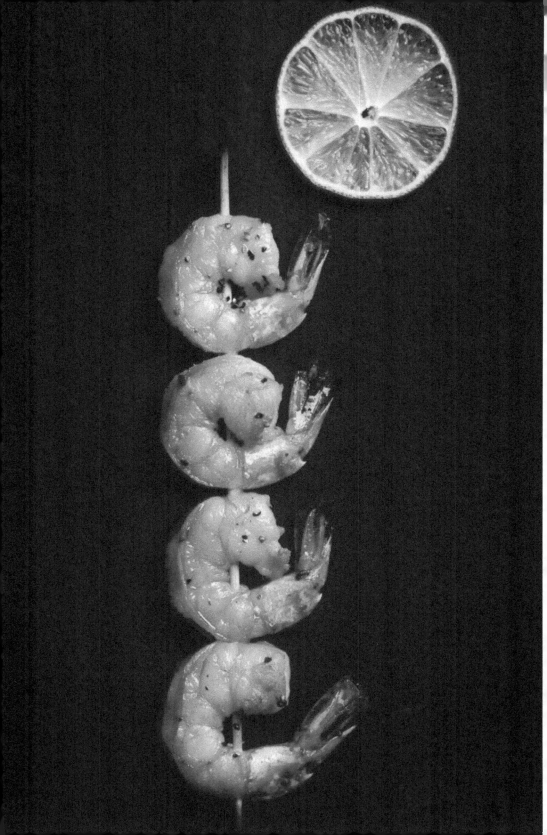

AMERICA'S RECIPES
——HUB——

—

4

Table of Contents

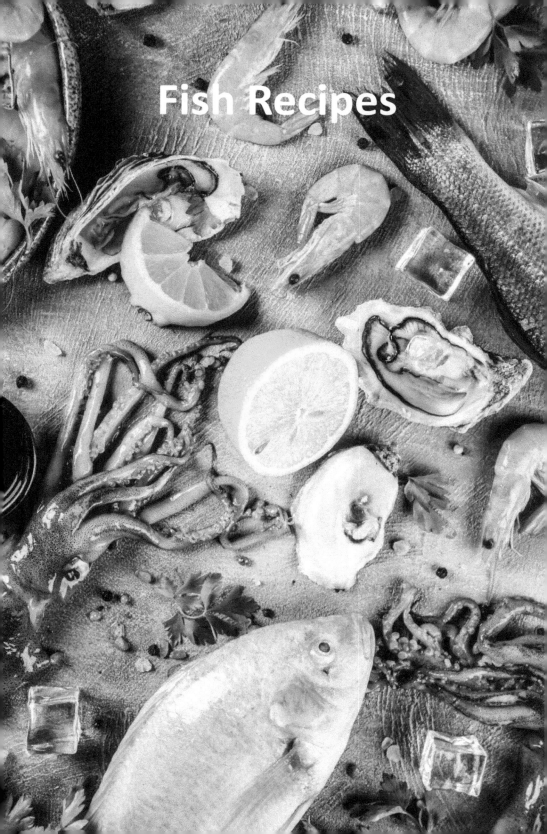

Fish Recipes

Cod with sautéed onions

4 servings | 15 minutes

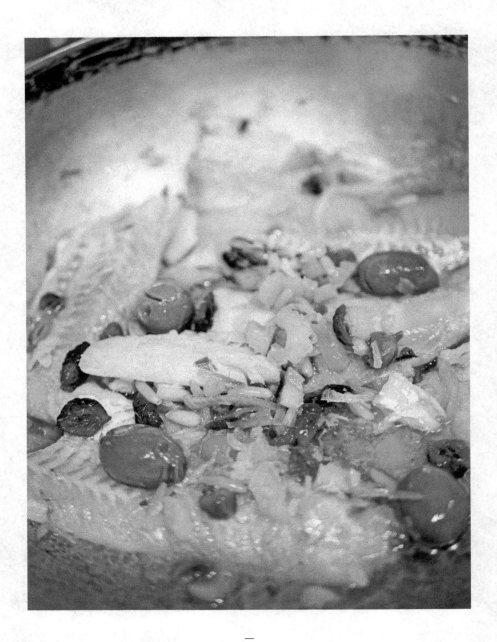

Ingredients:

1 lb. salt-tipped cod cut into pieces - 4 julienned onions - 8 garlic cloves - 1 julienned red pepper - Salt, pepper, bay leaf, and paprika - Boneless olives - Wheat flour - Olive oil - ½ cup sherry vinegar.

Instructions:

Preheat your Kalorik MAXX to 380°F by selecting the AIR FRY function. Meanwhile, flour the cod with salt and pepper on both sides.

Add the oil, onion, and garlic to the air fryer.
Insert the previously floured cod with pepper, bay leaf, paprika, and sherry vinegar. Cook for about 8 minutes, until golden brown.

In a large skillet, brown the garlic with the butter and olives over medium-low heat. Discard the garlic when sufficiently browned.

Transfer the cod with the onions to the skillet, add the lemon juice, and cook for an additional 4 minutes over high heat.

Place the cod on a serving platter and sprinkle with the mixture; serve immediately. Enjoy!

Foil Packet Salmon

2 Servings | 15 minutes

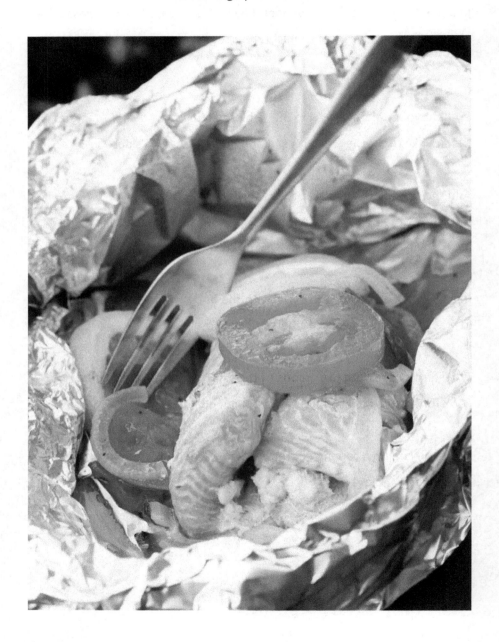

Ingredients:

2 x 4 oz skinless salmon fillets - 2 tbsp. unsalted butter, melted - ½ tsp. garlic powder - 1 medium lemon - ½ tsp. dried dill – 1 tomato

Instructions:

Take a sheet of aluminum foil and cut it into two squares measuring roughly 5" x 5". Lay each of the salmon fillets at the center of each piece.

Brush both fillets with a tablespoon of bullets and season with a quarter teaspoon of garlic powder.

Halve the lemon and grate the skin of one half over the fish. Cut four half-slices of lemon, using two to top each fillet. Season each fillet with a quarter-teaspoon of dill.

Fold the tops and sides of the aluminum foil over the fish to create a kind of packet. Place each one in the fryer.

Cook in your Kalorik MAXX for 10 minutes at 400°F. The salmon is ready when it flakes easily. Serve hot.

Monkfish In Almond Sauce

2 Servings | 15 minutes

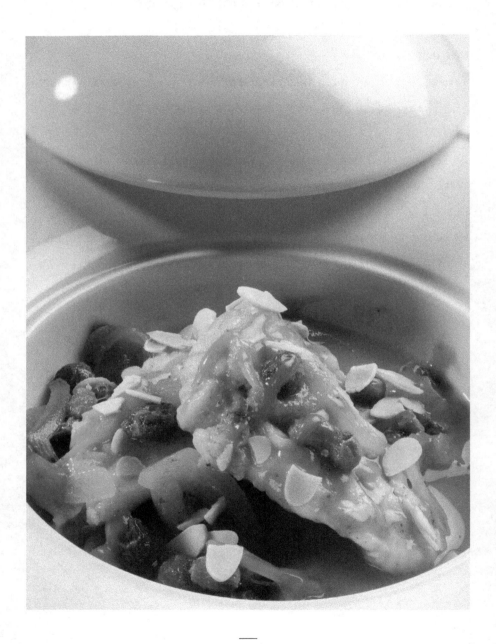

Ingredients:

A monk sliced into medallions. - Olive oil - 20 almonds - 3 garlic, mashed - 1 slice of bread in cubes - 1 cup of white wine - Salt and pepper - Laurel - Saffron - Wheat flour

Instructions:

Season the medallions, pass them through flour, take them to the Air Fryer painted with oil, and set them at 360ºc for 15-20 minutes.

Meanwhile, in a pan with olive oil, add the almonds and sauté. Add garlic, bread, and sauté.

Add 1 glass of water, wine, pepper, bay leaf, saffron, and salt to taste. Bring to a boil over low heat. Thicken and remove from heat.

Serve up the medallions with the sauce on top, and Serve up with mashed potatoes or rice.

Crusty Pesto Salmon

2 Servings | 15 minutes

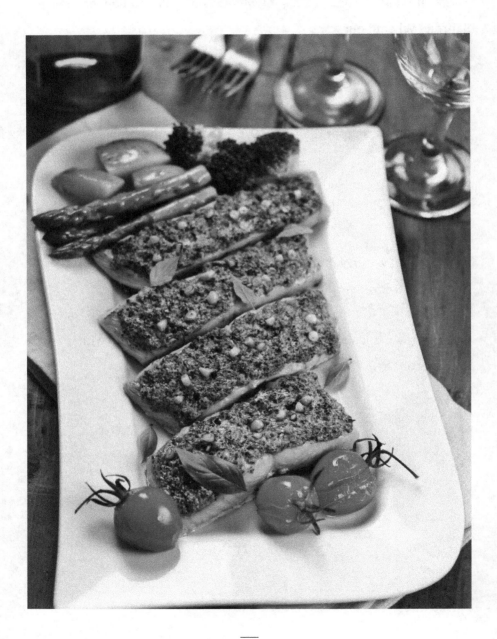

Ingredients:

¼ cup s, roughly chopped - ¼ cup pesto - 2 x 4 oz salmon fillets - 2 tbsp unsalted butter, melted

Instructions:

Mix the s and pesto together.

Place the salmon fillets in a round baking dish, roughly six inches in diameter.

Brush the fillets with butter, followed by the pesto mixture, ensuring to coat both the top and bottom. Put the baking dish inside the fryer.

Cook in your Kalorik MAXX for 12 minutes at 390°F.

The salmon is ready when it flakes easily when prodded with a fork. Serve warm.

Caramelized Prawns

4 Servings | 35 minutes

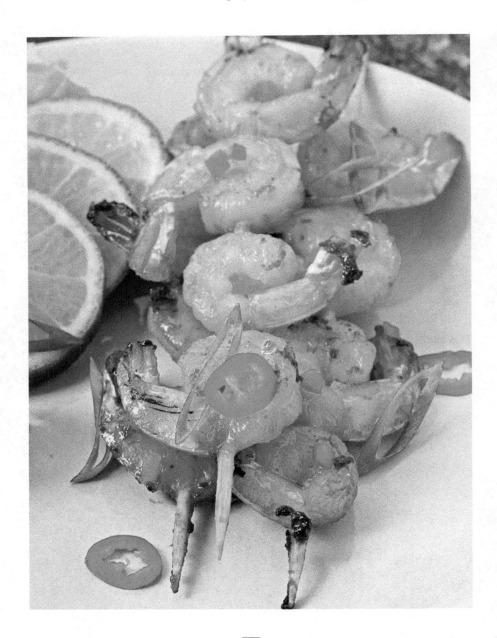

Ingredients:

24 clean prawns - Salt and pepper - Garlic and ginger - white wine - 4 oz carrot in canes - 8 oz julienne paprika - 4 oz purple onion julienne - 7 oz chives julienne - 1 avocado - Juice of 6 lemons - Olive oil - Teriyaki sauce

Instructions:

In a bowl, add the prawns, lemon juice, salt, and pepper.

Marinate in the refrigerator for 30 minutes. In the mold of your Kalorik MAXX, place oil and set it at 370ºC for 15 minutes.

At 5 minutes, add the prawns. 5 minutes later, add the wine and let it finish. Reserve up and cool.

In the same mold, add the vegetables and sauté at 350ºC for 12 minutes. Add garlic, ginger, salt, pepper, teriyaki, chives, and butter.

Add 5 minutes to finish the prawns. Serve up and decorate with avocado balls.

Crab Eggs

2 Servings | 15 minutes

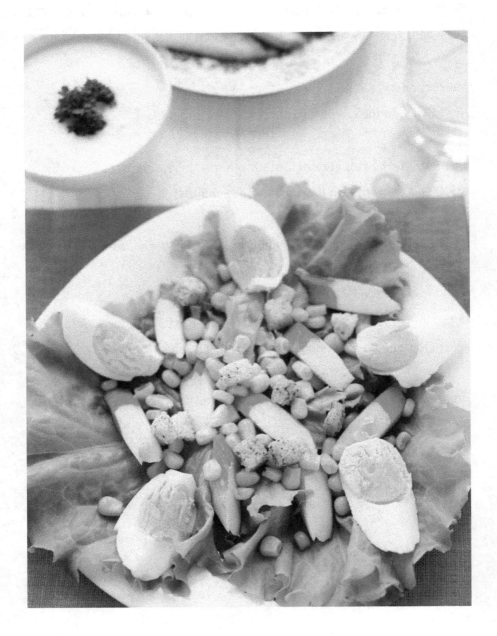

Ingredients:

1 pack of crab sticks

3 Eggs

1 Onion in small cubes

Red paprika in small cubes

Mustard - Olive oil –

cream cheese

1 lemon juice

Finely sliced coriander

Lettuce leaves

Instructions:

Place the eggs in a pot of water and boil for 12 minutes.

Remove, peel and cut in half. Remove the yolks and Reserve up. Crumble and cut the crab sticks.

Mix the yolks with oil, mustard, cheese, lemon, paprika, onion, and coriander.

Fill the whites with the mixture and Serve up on some lettuce leaves.

Tuna with Caper

3 Servings | 30 minutes

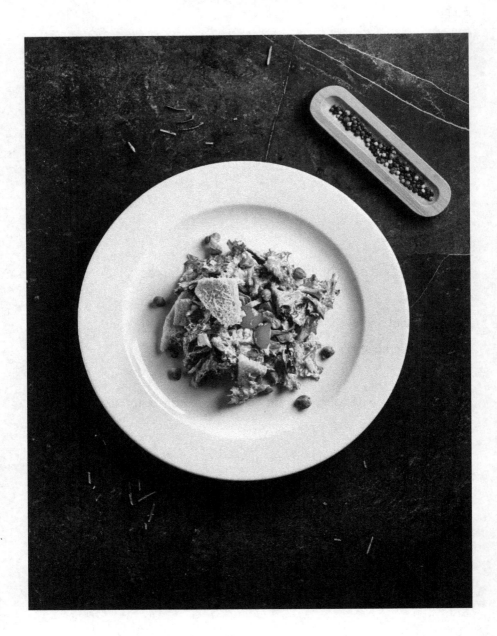

Ingredients:

8 oz Tuna

Olive oil

Salt and pepper

1 cup of mayonnaise

1 Natural yogurt

Finely chopped chive

1 tbsp of cut capers

1 Tablespoon mustard

Parsley finely cut

Instructions:

Season the tuna and bathe with olive oil. Sauté the chives and place them in a bowl.

Mix the chives, capers, mayonnaise, mustard, yogurt, and Reserve up.
Take the tuna to your Kalorik MAXX programmed at 370ºc for 10-18 minutes.

Halfway through flip, Serve up the tuna bathed with sauce and accompanied by pure or rice.

Crab Rolls

3 Servings | 30 minutes

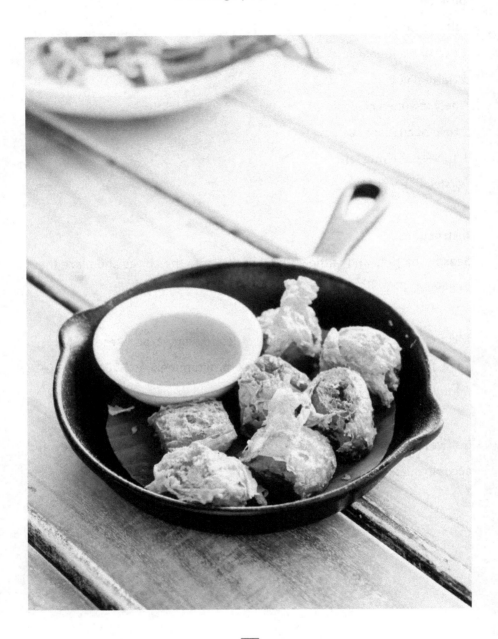

Ingredients:

2 paprika in julienne - Celery finely cut - ½ julienne zucchini - ½ carrot in canes - Soybean sprouts - Soy sauce - Finely sliced coriander - rice paper - Olive oil - Salt and pepper - Cut crab sticks - 4 orange juice - Vinegar – Sugar

Instructions:

In the mold of your Kalorik MAXX, set at 360°F for 15 minutes and add oil. At 5 minutes, add cereal, carrot, paprika, zucchini, and mix.

After 5 minutes, add sauce and soy beans. Mix and cook for 5 more minutes. Add coriander, mix, and Reserve up. Immerse the rice paper sheets until moistened.

Place the rice paper on film and place the stuffing and pieces of crab. Fold the side corners and seal the roll well.

Beat the passion fruit juice, olive oil, salt, sugar, pepper, and vinegar. Serve up the rolls and cover with the vinaigrette.

Raf Tomato with Prawns

2 Servings | 10 minutes

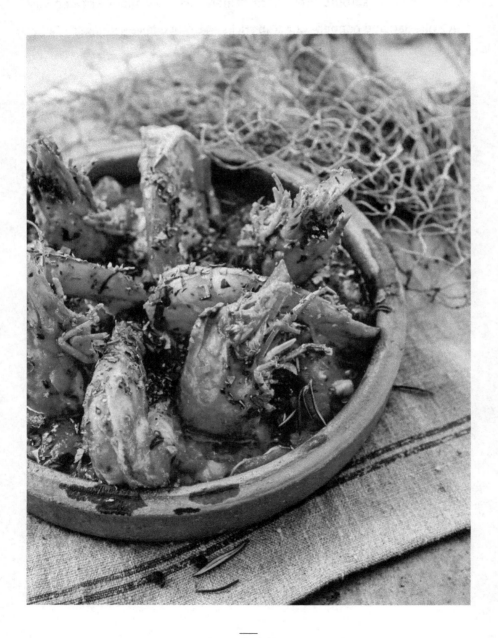

Ingredients:

2 raf tomatoes - 3 fl oz of Vegetable Broth - Olive oil - Parsley - 2 avocados (1 sliced) - Chardonnay vinegar - 1 chervil branch - 1 bunch of scallions - 1 spring onion julienne - 12 peeled - prawns – Salt

Instructions:

In the mold of the Kalorik MAXX, add hot water and prawns. Set at 370ºC for 1-4 minutes, cool in ice water, salt, and set aside.

Cut the tomatoes in 6 and season with salt, oil, and vinegar.
In a bowl, add the chopped avocado and mix with broth, salt, and oil. Grind, pass through a sieve, and Reserve.

Serve up, place the avocado cream on a plate, on top of it, the avocado in slices, prawns, tomato, chives, chervil, and chives. Season and bathe with oil.

Juicy Tuna Pie

4 Servings | 35 minutes

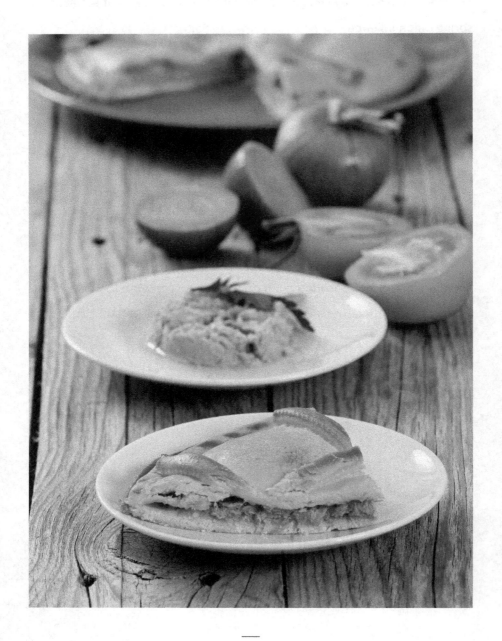

Ingredients:

10 oz Finely rounded onion - 2 kinds of garlic, mashed - 12 oz finely chopped paprika - Olive oil - 10 oz chopped tomato - Salt - 1 can of drained tuna - 3 Cooked eggs - 1 lb Wheat flour - Paprika - Instant yeast - Olive oil - White wine - 1 beaten egg

Instructions:

Sauté onion, garlic, and paprika until the color changes.

Add tomato, salt, sugar stir until thickened. Chop the tuna and mix with the chopped eggs.

Aside, mix flour, paprika, yeast, and salt. Add oil, wine, water, and mix until amalgamate. Let stand for 30 minutes.

Cut in 2 and stretch. Coat the mold of the Air Fryer with oil and cover with the dough. Fill with sautéing and tuna.

Cover with the other half of the dough, prick the surface, and seal the edges. Varnish with egg and set at 365°F for 20-25 minutes.

Cover with aluminum foil and reprogram for 15-20 minutes. Serve up hot.

Papillote Of White Fish

5 Servings | 20 minutes

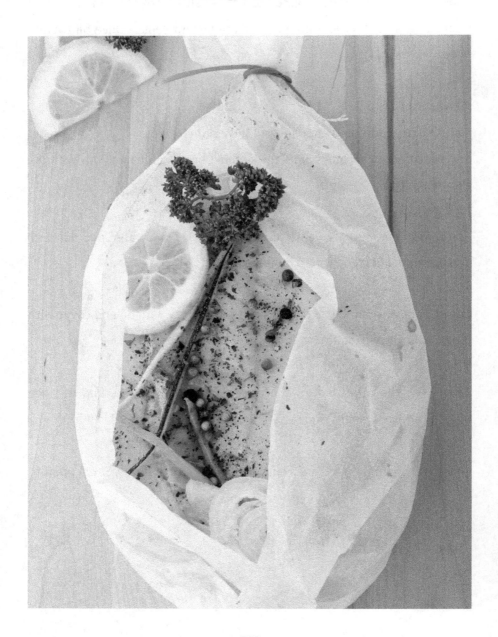

Ingredients:

8 white fish fillets - 1 rolled garlic - 1 lemon - 1 can of vegetables - 2 fish broth pellets - 3 oz of flour - Olive oil - Waxed paper

Instructions:

Cut the lemon in half, squeeze one half, and cut the other into slices.

Season the fillets with the shredded pastilles, Passthrough flour, and brown lightly in a pan with oil. Add garlic, lemon juice and reduce.

Take a rectangle of paper and place over 2 steaks. Add 2 tablespoons of vegetables, 1 slice of lemon, and a drizzle of oil. Close the paper like an envelope and seal.

Bring your Kalorik MAXX programmed at 365ºC for 10-15 minutes. Make an incision in the paper and Serve up by removing the inside of the envelope.

Fish with Paprika and Olives

2 Servings | 30 minutes

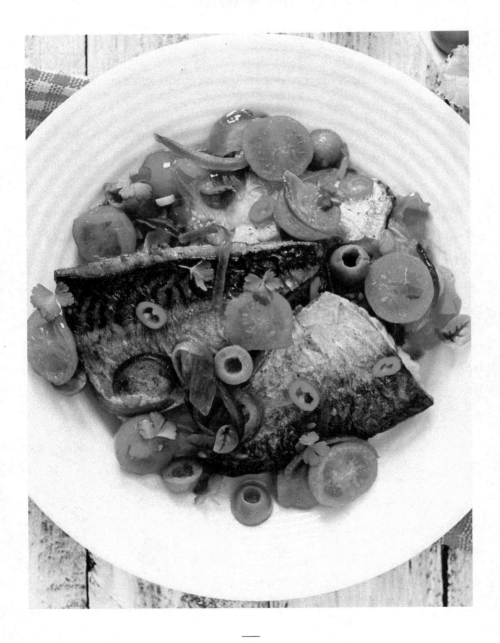

Ingredients:

2 White fish fillets - 1 Italian green paprika - 1 tomato - 1 garlic, mashed - 1 julienne onion - Stuffed Olives – Thyme - Olive oil - Salt and pepper

Instructions:

Process the tomato with garlic, oil, salt, and pepper.

Place aluminum foil in a pan and add the paprika until it turns black. Take it to a plastic bag and let it cool. Remove the skin, seeds and cut julienne.

On a sheet of aluminum foil, place tomato puree, top a steak, season, and season with thyme.

Cover with onion, paprika, and olives. Close and take the Air Fryer programmed at 3500ºc for 25 minutes. Serve up hot

Salmon Quiche and Leeks

3 Servings | 45 minutes

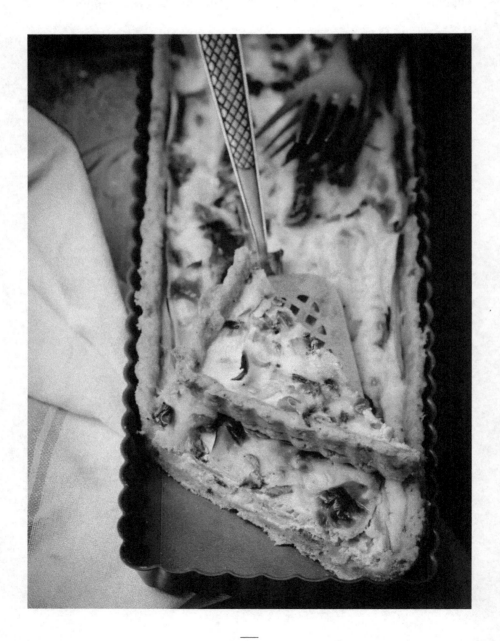

Ingredients:

1 sheet of dough breeze - 2 leeks - 4 oz of spinach. - 10 oz of fresh salmon. - 8 fl oz of milk - 4 fl oz of liquid cream - 3 eggs - Salt, pepper, nutmeg, and olive oil

Instructions:

Line the greased mold or lined with waxed paper with the dough. Seal with brushstrokes of the beaten egg.

Another sheet of paper is placed on top and brought to the Kalorik MAXX for 15-20 minutes per 350°F.

Lower and let stand. Take it without the paper that covered it before to the Air Fryer again for 6 minutes.

Cut into small pieces leeks and spinach, season and sauté. Apart, beat the eggs, cream, and place the milk, salt, and pepper, beat.

Add nutmeg and move. Distribute evenly over the dough; the leeks, spinach, and salmon. And cover with the previous mixture.

Take the Air Fryer for 15 minutes at a temperature of 350ºF

Tagliatelle with Salmon and Mirin Sauce

3 Servings | 30 minutes

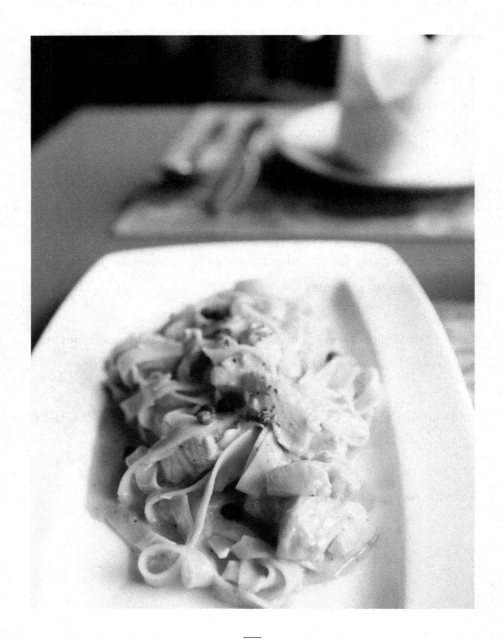

Ingredients:

10 oz Tagliatelle

8 oz salmon

2 oz toasted sesame seeds

Grated ginger

0.5 fl oz Rice vinegar

1 fl oz Soy sauce

Lemon juice

2 fl oz mirin sauce

Salt and pepper

Finely sliced coriander

Instructions:

Place in a bowl the sesame, ginger, rice vinegar, and mix.

Then add soy sauce, mirin, mix.

Line the mold of the Air Fryer with waxed paper and place the salmon.

Season and paint well with the sauce.

Schedule at 370°F for 15-20 minutes.

While cooking in boiling water with salt, the tagliatelle for 4 minutes.

Drain and add half of the sauce.

Serve up noodles in sauce with salmon and coriander.

Serve up the sauce separately.

Salmon with Leek and Teriyaki

4 Servings | 15 minutes

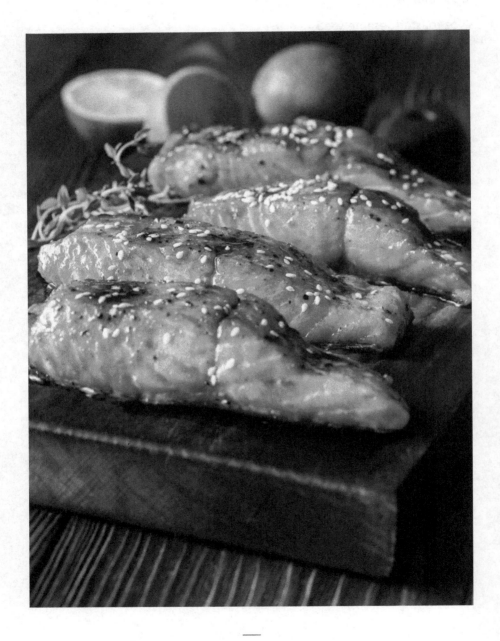

Ingredients:

4 salmon loins - 1 leek in julienne - 2 carrots in canes - 0.5 oz grated ginger - 4 tablespoons of teriyaki sauce - 4 tablespoons of port - 4 anise stars - Olive oil - Salt and pepper

Instructions:

Sauté leeks, carrots, and ginger until tender. In a double piece of aluminum foil, place a little of the vegetables and a spicy loin.

Cover with another bit of vegetable, add 1 tablespoon of teriyaki, port, and 1 anise star. Seal the envelope well and take the Air Fryer to 370ºC for 8-12 minutes.

Serve hot.

Russian Salmon Cake

5 Servings | 45 minutes

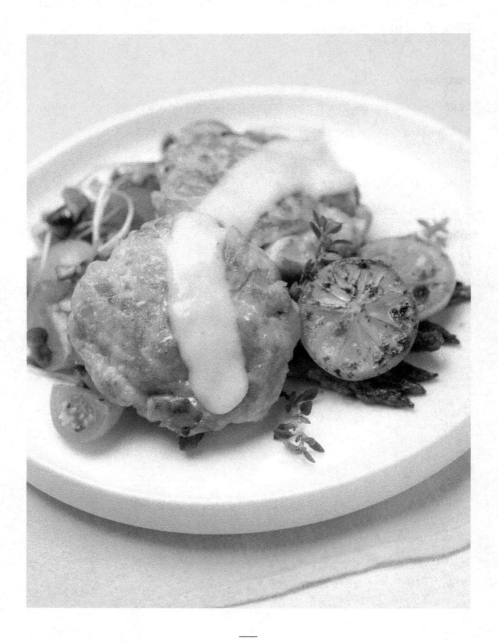

Ingredients:

12 oz Wheat flour - 10 oz Chopped butter - 1L Water - 4 Cooked eggs - 1 beaten egg - 1 oz Sunflower oil - 6 oz Long grain rice - 8 oz Onion - 1 garlic, mashed - 2 oz Butter - 10 oz Mushrooms - 1.5 lb Salmon clean - Salt and pepper - Finely cut dill

Instructions:

In the food processor, add flour, butter, salt, and mix. Then add 90ml of water and finish processing.

Make a ball, wrap with plastic wrap, and Reserve in the refrigerator for 30 minutes. Regularly make the rice and place it on a tray to cool. Grind garlic and onion in a blender.

Add butter, mushrooms and give small touches with the blender.

Place in a bowl, season, and Reserve up. Finely cut the eggs. Stretch the dough and place it in the mold of the Air Fryer wrapped in wax paper.

Fill with rice and on top of the mushrooms. Place the salmon and sprinkle with salt and dill.

Above all, place the eggs and cover them with more dough. Seal the edges, prick the dough, and brush with beaten egg.

Schedule your Kalorik MAXX at 370ºF for 20-25 minutes. Cover with aluminum foil and program for 10-12 minutes. Serve hot.

Shrimp Ceviche

5 Servings | 20 minutes

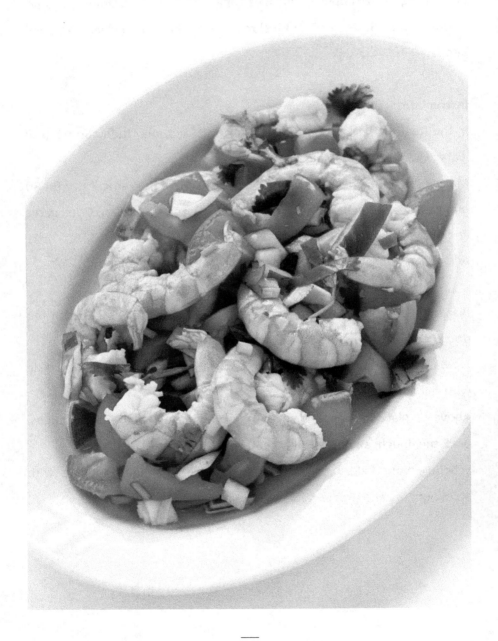

Ingredients:

2 lb of clean shrimp - 1 cup of lemon juice - 1 finely chopped onion - 2 finely chopped peppers - 2 tablespoons of tomato paste - Coriander and finely chopped basil - Salt and pepper

Instructions:

In a pot of water with boiling salt, place the shrimp until the color changes, drain and set aside. In the mold of the Air Fryer, add oil and set it at 350°F for 5 minutes.

Add onion, chili, coriander, and basil, mixing everything. Schedule at 320°F for 10 minutes, mixing every 5 minutes. Add the shrimp, tomato sauce, salt, and pepper, and mix well.

Serve up adding lemon, and accompany it with bread.

Salmon & Dill Sauce

2Servings | 30 minutes

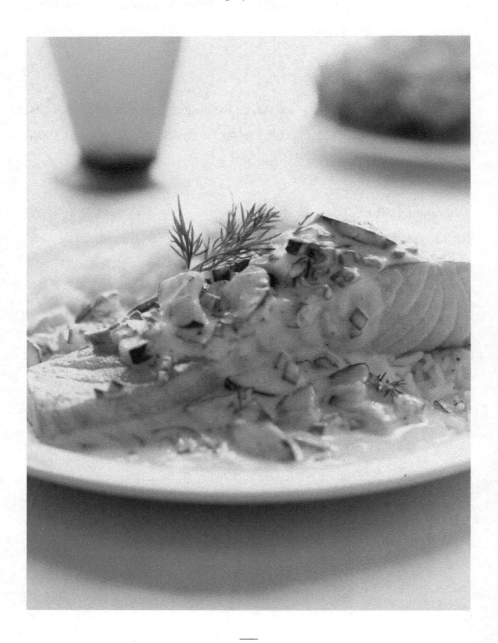

Ingredients:

For the Salmon:

1 ½ lb. salmon - 1 tsp. olive oil - 1 pinch salt

For the Dill Sauce:

½ cup non-fat Greek yogurt - ½ cup sour cream - Pinch of salt - 2 tbsp. dill, finely chopped

Instructions:

Select the AIR FRY function and preheat your Kalorik MAXX to 280°F.

Slice the salmon into four 6 oz. Pieces and pour a light drizzling of olive oil over each slice.

Sprinkle on the salt.

Put the salmon in the cooking basket and allow to cook for 20-23 minutes.

Prepare the dill sauce by mixing together the yogurt, sour cream, chopped dill, and salt.

Pour the sauce over the salmon and top with another sprinkling of chopped dill before serving.

Octopus with Broccoli

4 Servings | 45 minutes

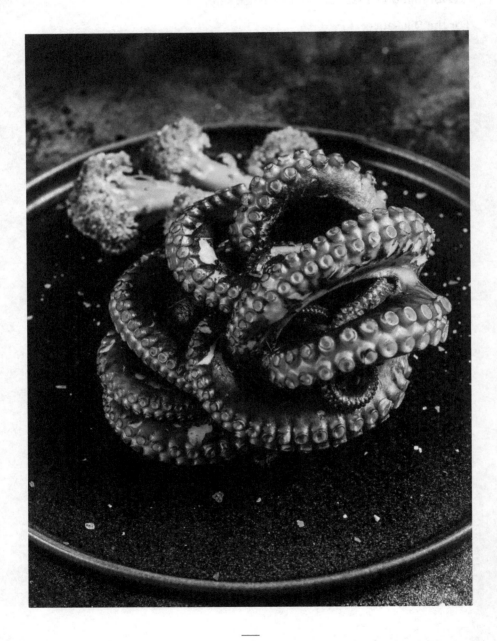

Ingredients:

1 clean octopus – 1 lb small potatoes - 3 cloves of garlic, mashed - Parsley finely cut - Olive oil - port wine - green olives without bone - Salt and pepper in grains - 2 eggs - Broccoli shelled

Instructions:

In a pot of boiling water, with salt and pepper, soak the octopus several times to "scare" it and leave it inside for 10 minutes.

Apart from boiling water with salt, place the potatoes for 10 minutes. In another pot with water, add the eggs and boil count 10 minutes, remove and reserve.

In that water, add the broccoli for 3 minutes and Reserve up.
Cut the tentacles of the octopus. Cover the Air Fryer's mold with oil, add the octopus, top the potatoes, parsley, garlic, salt, and pepper, add the olives, and cover everything with the port and oil.

Program the Kalorik MAXX at 350ºF for 15-20 minutes. Meanwhile, cut and mix the eggs and broccoli.
Serve up the octopus together with the broccoli.

Sunday's Salmon

3 Servings | 20 minutes

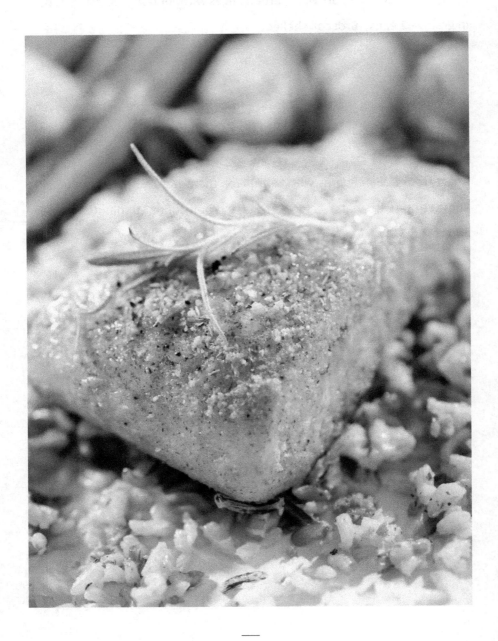

Ingredients:

½ lb. salmon fillet, chopped - 2 egg whites - 2 tbsp. Chives, chopped - 2 tbsp. garlic, minced - ½ cup onion, chopped - 2/3 cup carrots, grated - 2/3 cup potato, grated - ½ cup friendly bread crumbs - ¼ cup flour - Pepper and salt

Instructions:

In a shallow dish, combine the bread crumbs with pepper and salt.

Pour the flour into another dish. In a third dish, add the egg whites.

Put all of the other ingredients in a large mixing bowl and stir together to combine.

Using your hands, shape equal amounts of the mixture into small balls. Roll each ball in the flour before dredging it in the egg, and lastly covering it with bread crumbs. Transfer all the coated croquettes to the Kalorik MAXX and air fry at 360°F for 6 minutes.

Reduce the heat to 320°F and allow to cook for another 4 minutes. Serve hot.

Tilapia Fillets

3 Servings | 25 minutes

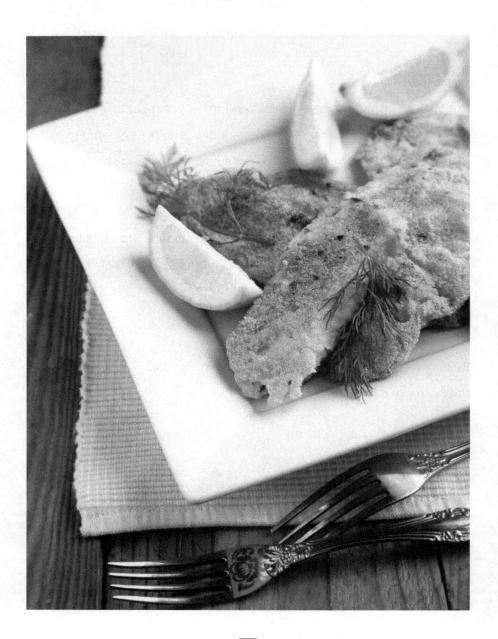

Ingredients:

1 lb. tilapia fillets, sliced

4 wheat buns

2 egg yolks

1 tbsp. fish sauce

2 tbsp. mayonnaise

3 sweet pickle relish

1 tbsp. hot sauce

Instructions:

In a bowl, mix together the egg yolks and fish sauce.

Throw in the mayonnaise, sweet pickle relish, and hot sauce.

Transfer the mixture to a round baking tray.

Put it in the Kalorik MAXX and line the sides with the tilapia fillets.

Cook for 15 minutes at 300°F.

Remove and serve on hamburger buns if desired.

Catfish Fillets Special

3 Servings | 20 minutes

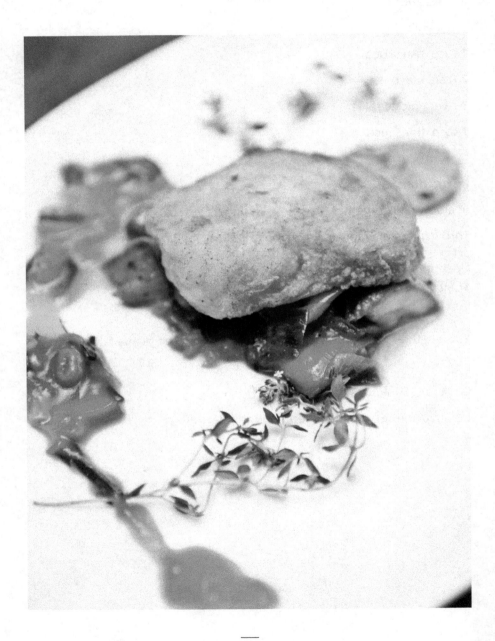

Ingredients:

2 catfish fillets - 1 teaspoon of ginger – 2 oz of butter - 4 oz of Worcestershire sauce - 1 cubicle jerk seasoning - 1 mustard casserole - 1 spoonful of balsamic vinegar - ½ cup of Catsup - Salt and black chili - 1 spoonful of parsley, chopped

Instructions:

Heat a skillet over medium heat with the butter, add Worcestershire seasoning of sauce, garlic, mustard, catsup, vinegar, salt, and hot pepper. Adjust fire, swirl well, and apply fish fillets.

Toss well, leave the fillets for 10 minutes, drain them, pass them to the preheated Kalorik MAXX oven.

Cook at 350° F for 10 minutes. Divide into bowls, brush on top with parsley and serve immediately. Enjoy!

Tasty Red Snapper

4 Servings | 45 minutes

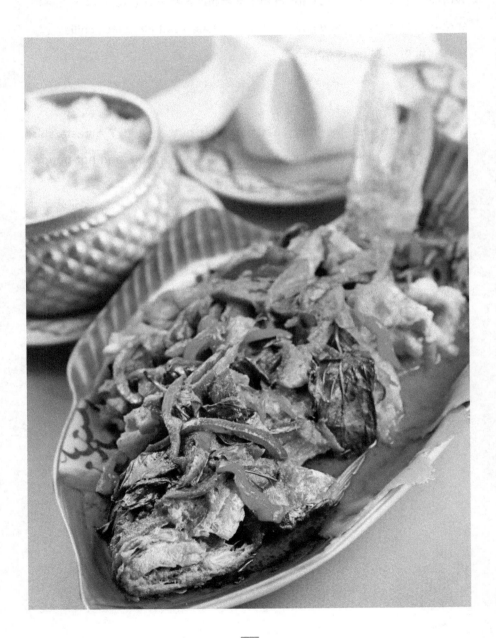

Ingredients:

1 wide red snapper, tidy and scored - Salt and black chili, to try - 3 cloves of garlic, minced - 1 jalapeno, split - 0.5 lb of okra, hacked - 1 tbsp of butter - 2 tbsp of olive oil - 1 chopped red bell pepper - 2 Spoonful of white wine

Instructions:

Mix jalapeno, wine, and garlic in a cup. Stir well, season with salt and pepper, and cook for 30 minutes.

Meanwhile, turn on the Kalorik MAXX 1 tablespoon butter, add the pepper and okra mix, and cook for 5 minutes.

Fill the belly of the red snapper with this combination, introduce the parsley and rub with olive oil.

Place in the AirFryer and cook for fifteen minutes at 400°F, turning the fish halfway through cooking

Stuffed Calamari

4 Servings | 30 minutes

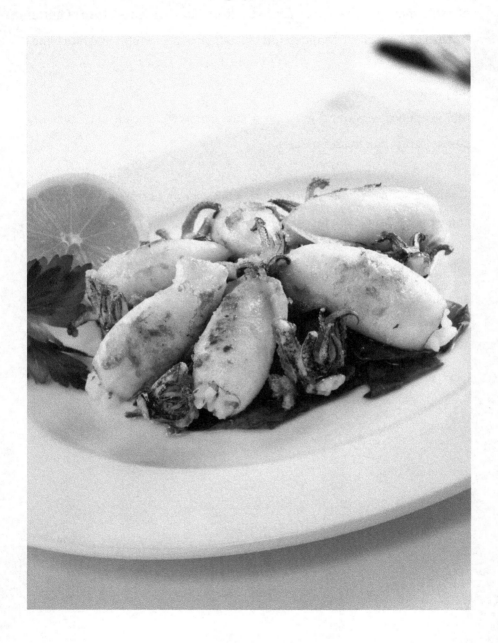

Ingredients:

4 giant calamari, split and sliced tentacles, and allocated tubes - 2 tablespoons of parsley, chopped - 5 ounces of kale, chopped - 2 cloves of garlic, minced - 1 chopped red bell pepper - 1 tsp of olive oil - 2 ounces of canned tomato puree - 1 yellow onion, sliced - Salt and black chili

Instructions:

Preheat a saucepan over medium pressure, incorporate onion and garlic. Cook for 2 minutes to combine and prepare.

Insert the pepper bell, the tomato puree, the tentacles of calamari, the spinach, salt, and stir in pepper, cook for 10 minutes, then take off fire. Stir in, and cook for three minutes.

Stuff calamari tubes with this combination, placed in healthy with toothpicks. Cook for 20 minutes at 360°F.
Divide calamari into bowls, scatter with parsley and serve. Enjoy!

Lemon and Fish Relish

2 Servings | 40 minutes

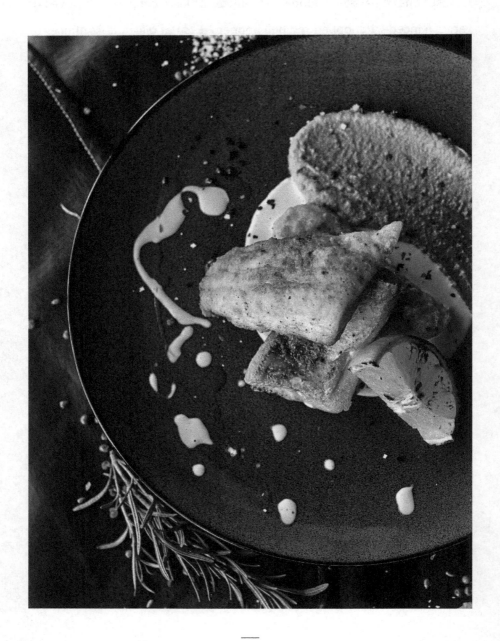

Ingredients:

2 salmon fillets, boneless - Salt and black chili, to satisfy - 1 tbsp of olive oil - 1 tsp lemon juice - 1 shallot, cut - 1 lemon, diced and cut into wedges - Olive oil

Instructions:

Season salmon with salt and pepper, fried with 1 cubic cubicle of oil. Put it in the basket of your Kalorik MAXX and cook at 320°F for 20 minutes halfway, tossing the fish.

Meanwhile, blend shallot and lemon juice in a cup, a sprinkle of salt and black pepper, and keep on for ten min.
Mix the marinated shallot in a different bowl with the lemon slices, salt, parsley, pepper, and oil, and shake well.

Divide salmon into bowls, relish and serve top with citrus. Enjoy!

Salmon Orange

4 Servings | 10 minutes

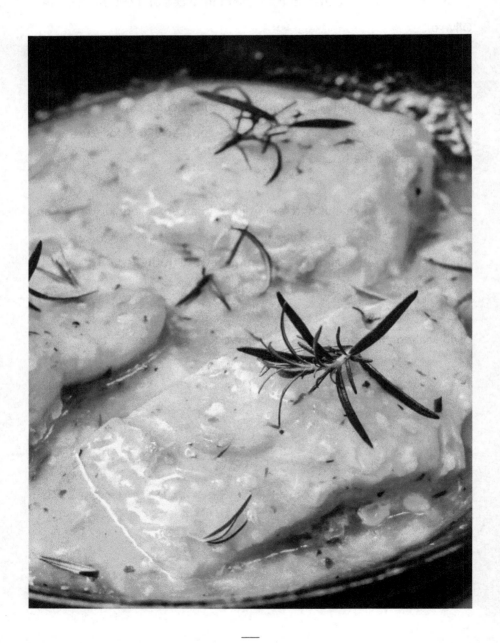

Ingredients:

1 lb of wild salmon, skinless, ossified, and cubed - 2 cut lemons - ¼ cup of Balsamic vinegar - ¼ tablespoon of orange juice - ¼ tablespoon of orange marmalade - A tablespoon of black pepper and salt

Instructions:

Heat the vinegar in a pot over medium pressure, add marmalade, and the orange juice, stir, simmer for 1 minute and bring to a boil. Let it off.

Cut salmon and slices of lemon on skewers, season with salt, rub them with half the orange marmalade and black pepper. Mix, put in the basket of your Kalorik MAXX, cook at 360°F for 3 minutes.

Pinch skewers with most of the vinegar mixture, divided between, cover with a side salad, and serve promptly. Enjoy!

Mustard Salmon

1 Serving | 15 minutes

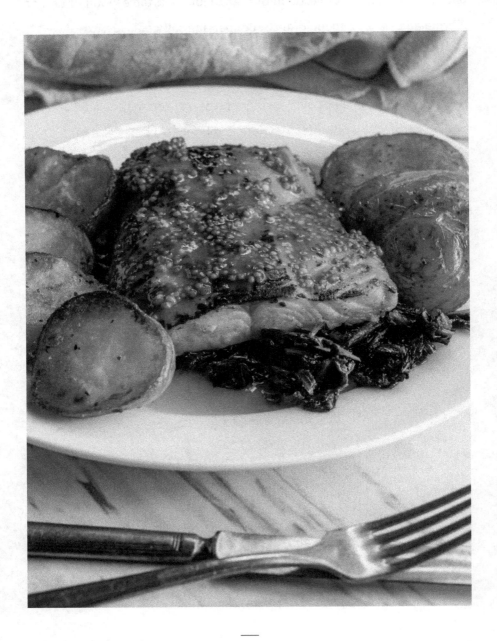

Ingredients:

1 boneless salmon fillet

Salt and black chili

2 mustard spoons

1 tsp of coconut oil

1 tbsp of maple

Instructions:

Mix the maple extract and mustard in a tub, whisk well, season well the salmon with salt and pepper, and salmon brown with this combination.

Sprinkle some cooking spray over fish, put it in the Kalorik MAXX, and cook 10 minutes at 370°F, turning in half.

Serve with a flavorful salad on the side. Enjoy!

Italian Barramundi Fillets

4 Servings | 20 minutes

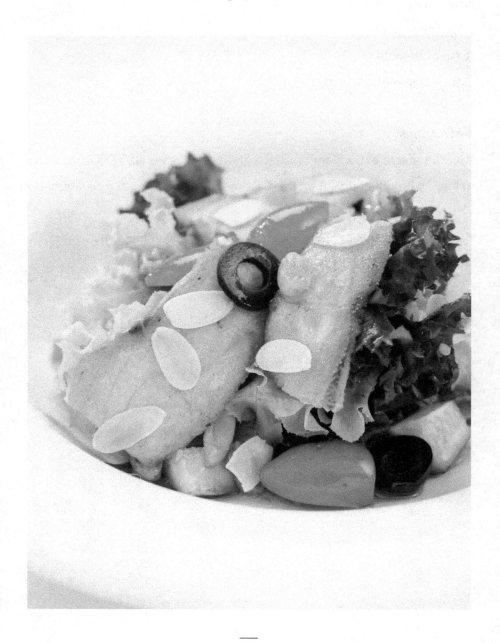

Ingredients:

2 barramundi, boneless fillets - Olive oil - 2 Italian seasoning teaspoons green olives, diced and pitted - ½ cup cherry tomatoes, chopped - ½ cup of black olives - 1 lemon zest - 2 lemon zest spoons - Salt and black chili - 2 tsp parsley, chopped

Instructions:

Apply salt, pepper, Italian seasoning, and 2 teaspoons of olive oil. Transfer the oil to your Kalorik MAXX and cook for 8 minutes at 360° F, halfway, tossing them.

Mix the tomatoes in a dish with black olives, green olives, salt, pepper, lemon zest, lemon juice, parsley, and 1 tbs of olive oil. Toss well.

Divide the fish into bowls, fill with tomato salsa and Enjoy!

Shrimps and Crabs Mix

4 Servings | 30 minutes

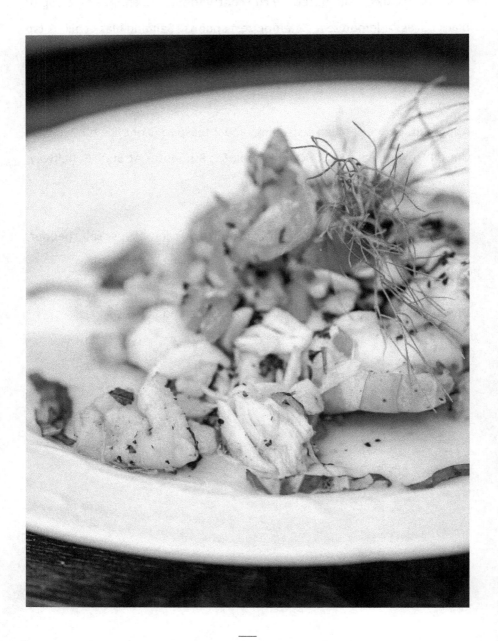

Ingredients:

1 cup of yellow, minced onion - 1 cup of green potatoes, diced - 1 cup of celery, cut - 1 pound of crawls, sliced - 1 cup of crabmeat, sliced - 1 cup of mayonnaise - 1 Worcestershire teaspoon sauce - Salt and black chili, to try - 2 tablespoons of sliced bread - 1 tablespoon of butter, melted - 1 tablespoon of tender paprika

Instructions:

Comb shrimp and crab meat in a dish, bell pepper, tomato, mayo, sauce with celery, garlic, chili pepper, and Worcestershire, mix well, and pass to the casserole that suits your fryer.

Sprinkle the crumbs and the paprika with the crust, apply the melted butter and put in your Kalorik MAXX, and bake for 25 minutes at 320° F, midway. Divide between bowls and serve immediately. Enjoy!

Asian Halibut

3 Servings | 40 minutes

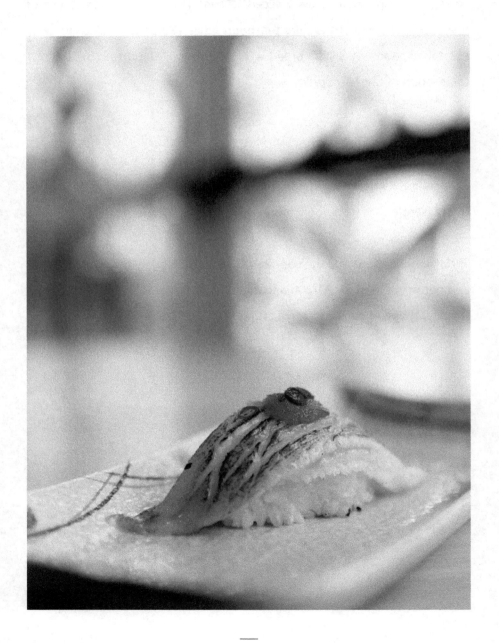

Ingredients:

1 lb of halibut steaks - 1 fl oz Soy sauce - 1 spoonful of sugar - 2 spoonfuls of lime juice - ½ teaspoon red pepper flakes - ½ tablespoon of orange juice - ½ tablespoon of ginger powder, grated - 1 clove of garlic, minced

Instructions:

Place soy sauce in a saucepan, fire over a moderate flame, including mirin, sugar, lime and orange juice, ginger and garlic, pepper flakes, blend well. Bring it to a boil, and heat off.

Put half of the marinade in a cup, add halibut, toss to cover, then leave them in the refrigerator for 30 minutes.

Switch the halibut to the Kalorik MAXX and cook for 10 minutes at 390° F, only flipping once.

Divide halibut steaks into bowls, scatter with the rest of the marinade. Serve and enjoy!

Wrapped Shrimps

6 Servings | 20 minutes

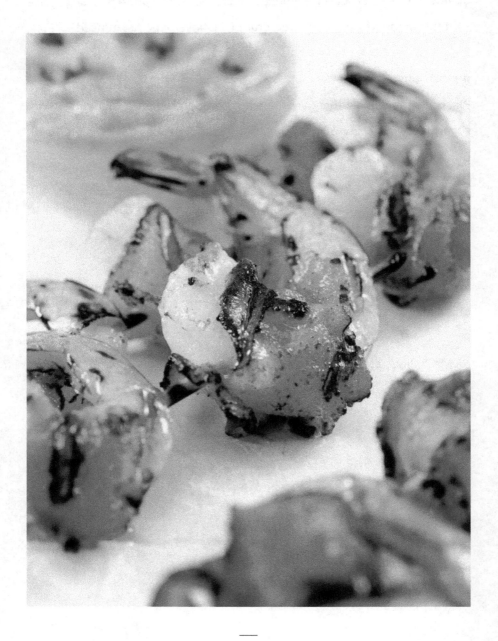

Ingredients:

1 fl oz of olive oil - 10 oz of shrimp already baked, peeled, and deveined - 1 spoonful basil, minced - ¼ cups of blackberries, ground – 10 slices prosciutto - red wine

Instructions:

Wrap a slice of prosciutto, drizzle over the oil, cut well, but it at 390° F in your Kalorik MAXX and fry them for 8 minutes.

In the meantime, fire up a saucepan with blackberries over medium heat, add mint and juice, stir, simmer for three minutes, then turn off.

Place shrimp on a tray, sprinkle blackberry sauce over them and serve as an appetizer.

Appetizer of Cajun Shrimp

3 Servings | 10 minutes

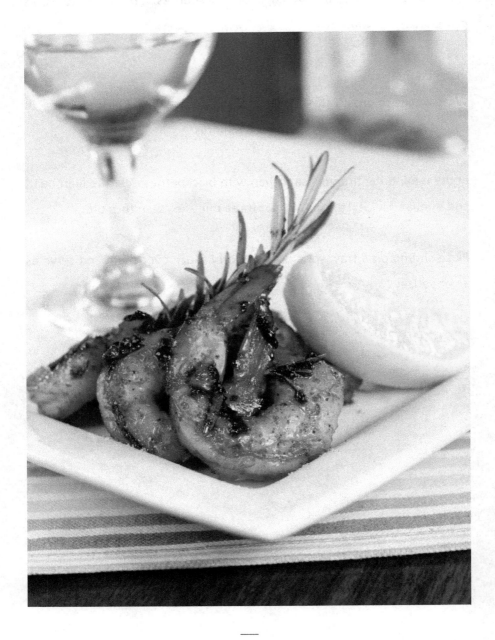

Ingredients:

20 tiger shrimps, peeled

Salt and black chili, to satisfy

Seasoning with ½ teaspoon of the old bay

1 tablespoon of olive oil

¼ smoked paprika teaspoon

Instructions:

Comb the shrimps in a bowl with the salt, pepper, old bay seasoning, paprika, and toss to coat.

Place the shrimp in the basket of your Air Fryer and cook at 390°F for 5 minutes.

Put them up on a tray and serve as an appetizer. Enjoy!

Chips and Fish

2 Servings | 20 minutes

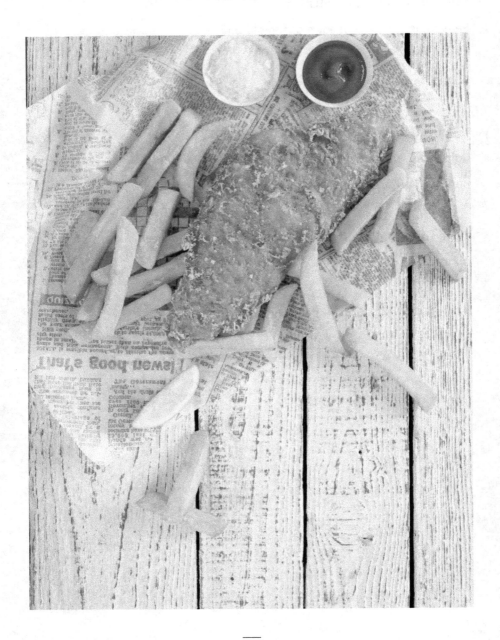

Ingredients:

2 medium fillets of char, skinless and osseous - Salt and black chili - ¼ cup of buttermilk - 3 cups of the kettle, fried chips

Instructions:

Mix fish with salt, pepper, and buttermilk in a tub, then mix and set aside 5 minutes. Place chips and grind them in the mixing bowl and scatter them on a tray.

Add fish and push both sides tight. Switch fish to the basket of your Kalorik MAXX and cook at 400°F for 12 minutes. For lunch, serve hot.

Fish Club Sandwich

2 Servings | 40 minutes

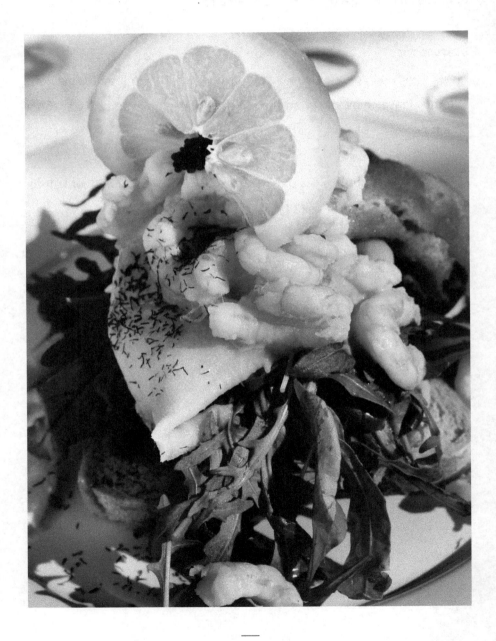

Ingredients:

2 slices of whole white bread

1 tbsp of smooth butter

1 tin of tuna

1 little capsicum

For Barbeque sauce:

¼ tbsp of Worcestershire - ½ tbsp of olive oil - ½ crushed garlic flake - ¼ cup of sliced onion - ¼ tsp of powdered mustard - ½ tbsp of Zucker - ¼ tbsp of red sauce chili - 1 tbsp of ketchup tomatoes - A sprinkle of salt and black chilies to taste

Instructions:

Pick the bread slices and cut the rims. Now clean the slices in the horizontal context. Heat the sauce ingredients and wait until the sauce thickens. Now fill in the catch the sauce and whisk until the flavors are obtained. Whisk the capsicum and roast, peel off the skin. The capsicum is cut into chunks and add it to slices of bread.

Heat up the Kalorik MAXX to 300°F for five minutes. Open the basket of the fryer and put the sandwiches in it. Now hold the fryer at 250° F for fifteen minutes.

Flip the sandwiches in-between the process of preparation. Serve the sandwiches with tomato ketchup or mint chutney.

Crispy Tempura Shrimps

2 Servings | 30 minutes

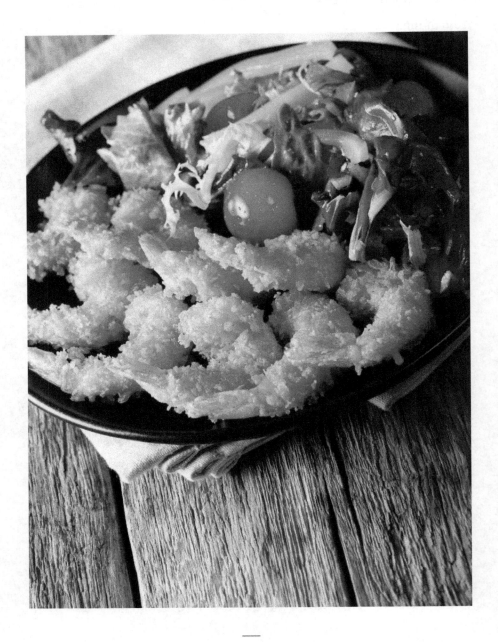

Ingredients:

6 oz of flour tempura - 6 oz of water - 4 oz of tiger shrimp

Instructions:

Transfer water to tempura flour and blend with a whisk. Peel off the shell shrimp but don't cut the tail. Cut the back and cut the esophagus.

Create incisions inside the curve. Switch over and press the back before you spread the shrimp.
Drain shrimp and pepper.

Place the shrimps in the flour for the tempura and dive in the butter.
Then cook for 2 minutes at a temperature of 170°F in deep-frying. Place the prawns on towels made from paper.

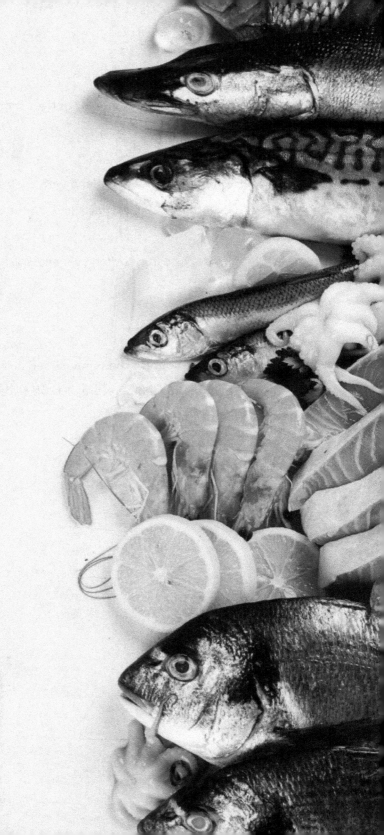

Salads & Side Dishes

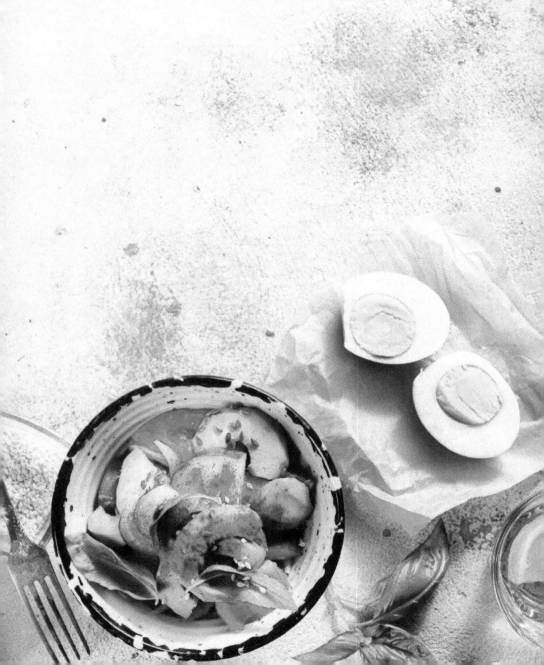

Seabass Salad

3 Servings | 25 minutes

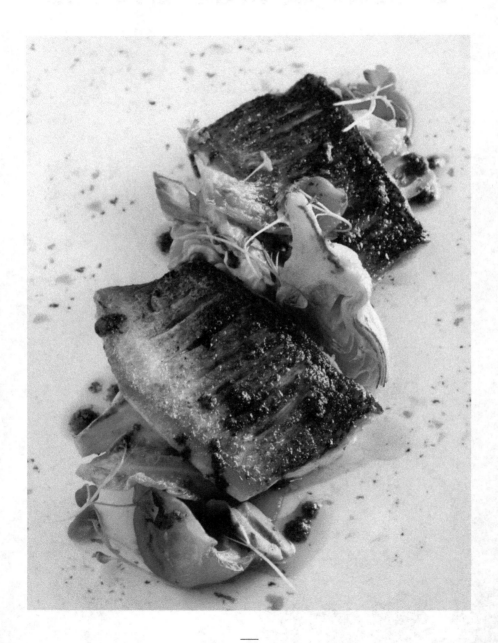

Ingredients:

7 oz of salad - 1 tablet of Fish Paella - Olive oil - 2 clean sea bass - 1 lemon sliced - Salt, Pepper, Rosemary, and Salvia

Instructions:

Fill the sea bass with lemon, sage, and rosemary. Season with salt on the outside and place on aluminum foil.

To season with the crumbled tablet, a splash of oil, and to close the aluminum foil.

Bring the Kalorik MAXX programmed at 390°F for 10 minutes. File the fish and Serve up with salad.

Bites Fried Tuna Salad

3 Servings | 20 minutes

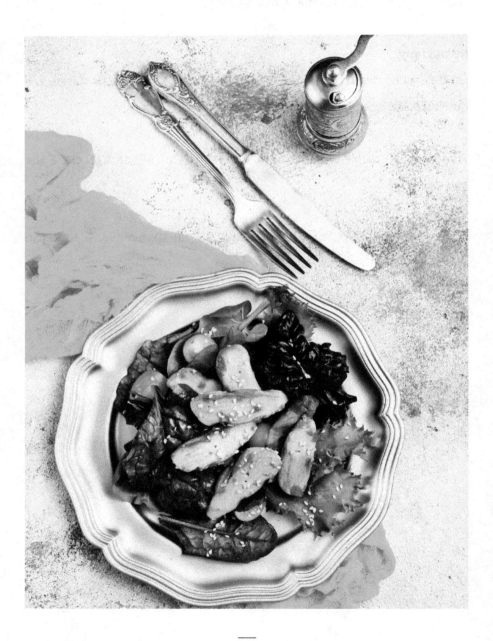

Ingredients:

10 oz of drained tuna - ¼ cup of full-bodied mayonnaise - 1 celery stalk chopped - 1 strong, sliced, pitted, and mashed avocado - ¼ cup of finely blanched almond flour, break - 2 tsp of coconut oil

Instructions:

Combine the tuna, mayonnaise, celery, and a large bowl, mix the avocado mashed in. Form the blend into balls.

Roll balls of coconut oil in almond flour and spritz—place balls in the Kalorik MAXX basket.

Set the temperature to 400° F, then set the timer to 7 Minutes. Switch the tuna bites softly over after 5 minutes. Serve hot.

Fisherman's salad

2 servings | 10 minutes

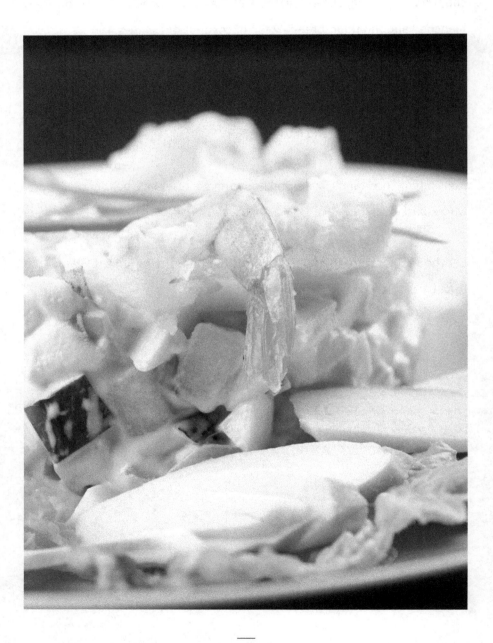

Ingredients:

4 fried shrimp - 4 ounces fried cod - 2 julienned onions - 2 julienned bell peppers - 1 julienned zucchini - Olive oil - 3 oz lettuce - Soy sauce - Salt & pepper

Introductions:

In a large bowl, add the fish, soy sauce, salt and pepper, garlic, and a drizzle of olive oil.

Stir and let marinate for 5 minutes.

Take the air fryer and place the fish and marinade in.

Set at 340°F for 8 minutes.

When cooked through, remove the fish.

Add the oil and sauté the onions with the remaining cooking liquid.

Stir the resulting compounds into the zucchini, peppers, and fish. Serve the salad and drizzle with the sauce.

Salmon Lettuce Blend

3 servings | 10 minutes

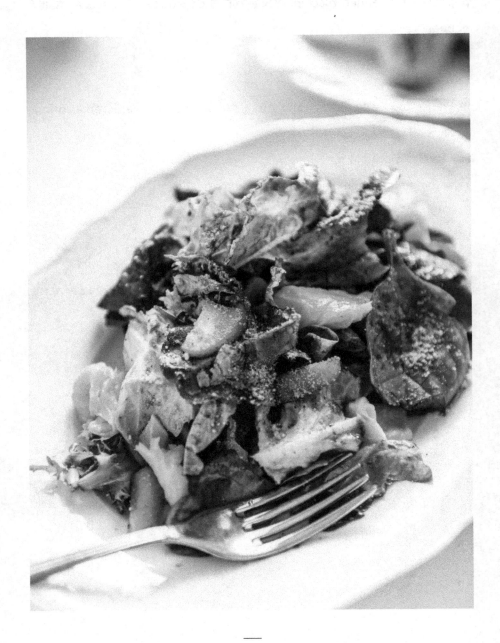

Ingredients:

Lettuce - 4 tablespoons olive oil - 8 ounces salmon fillets, skinless and boneless - Salt and pepper - 1 tablespoon chives, chopped - 1 tablespoon parsley, chopped - 1 tablespoon fresh tarragon, chopped - 3 tablespoons shallots, chopped - 1 lemon zest rubbed into a cube - 1/4 cup juice of one lemon

Instructions:

Mix lettuce with 1/2 cubic tablespoon oil in a bowl and swirl to coat. Sprinkle with salt and pepper; place on a baking sheet.
Place the salmon in the Kalorik MAXX at 450°F and bake for 5 minutes.

Combine the chives with the parsley and tarragon in a bowl, then sprinkle 1 cube over the salmon.

Meanwhile, toss with the lemon juice and the rest of the herbs, and blend well. Add 2 tablespoons of the shallots to the mixed greens and toss gently.
Remove salmon from oven, set aside on bowls, add greens. Drizzle the remaining shallot dressing over the side and serve immediately.

Avocado Salad

2 Servings | 15 minutes

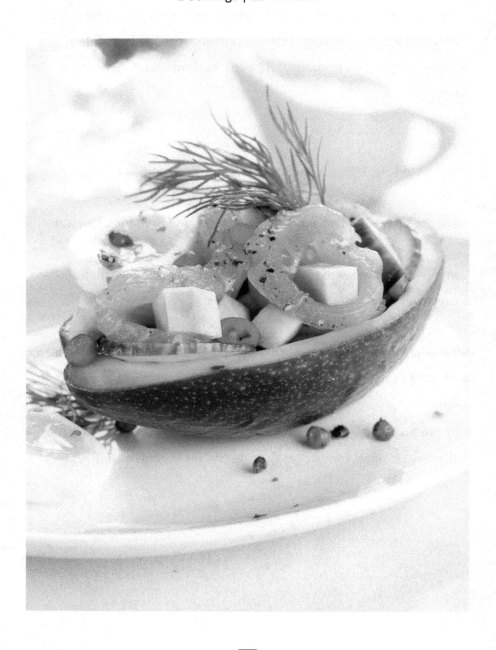

Ingredients:

2 fried cod fillets - 4 hard egg yolks - 6 peeled prawns - 1 avocado in cubes - 1 paprika roasted in cubes- 6 pickled cucumbers (cubed) - Chopped capers - Olive oil

Instructions:

In the Air Fryer, place the prawns and cod with a bit of oil, season, and set at 375°F for 5-8 minutes.

Apart, mix avocado, pickles, yolks, capers, paprika, and season with oil, pepper, and the shredded tablet.

Serve up a bed of salad, top the prawns, and garnish with the eggs.

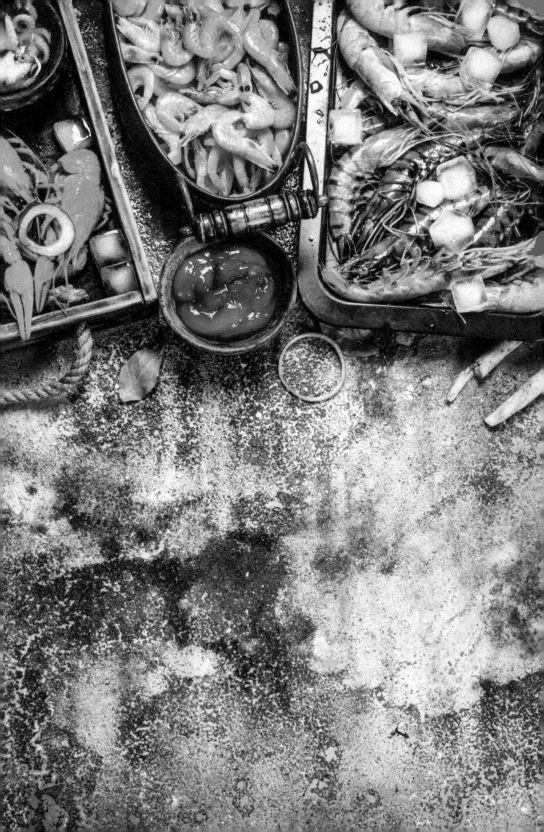

BAKERY & PASTRY

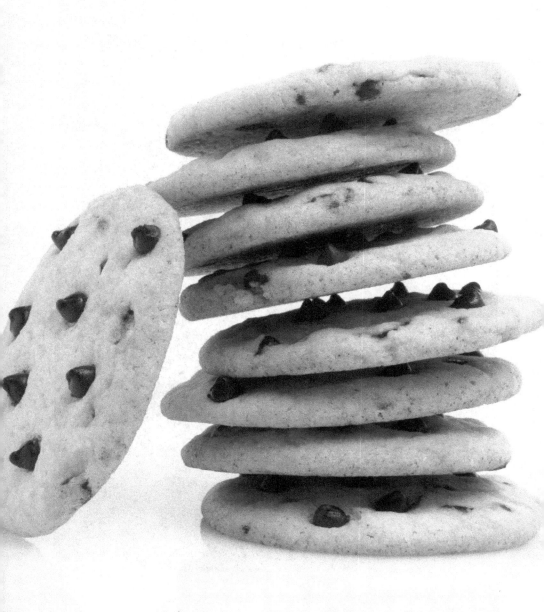

Air Fry Choco Cookies

8 Servings | 35 minutes

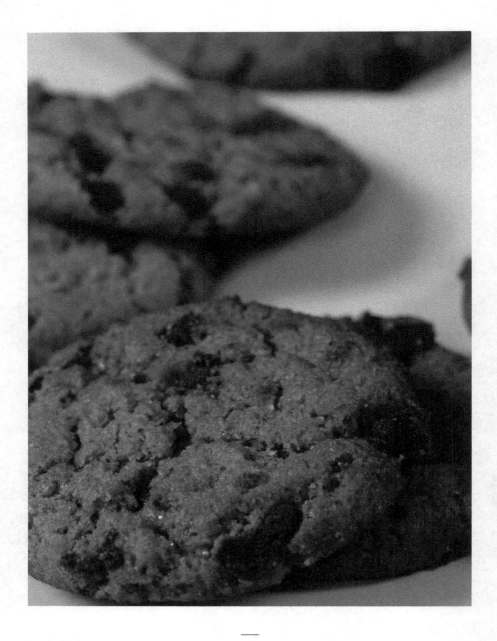

Ingredients:

1 teaspoon of vanilla extract - Half cup of butter - 1 egg - Four spoonfuls of sugar - 2 cups of flour - 1⁄2 cup of unsweetened chocolate chips

Instructions:

Heat butter in a saucepan over medium pressure, stir, and cook for 1 minute. Comb egg and vanilla extract with sugar in a cup, then mix well.

Stir in butter, flour, and half of the chocolate chips and stir all.
Move this to a saucepan that suits your fryer and disperse the rest of the chocolate chips on top, introduce it in the fryer at 300° F.

Bake for another 25 minutes. Slice when cold, and then serve. Enjoy it!

Maple Cinnamon Buns

9 Servings | 50 minutes

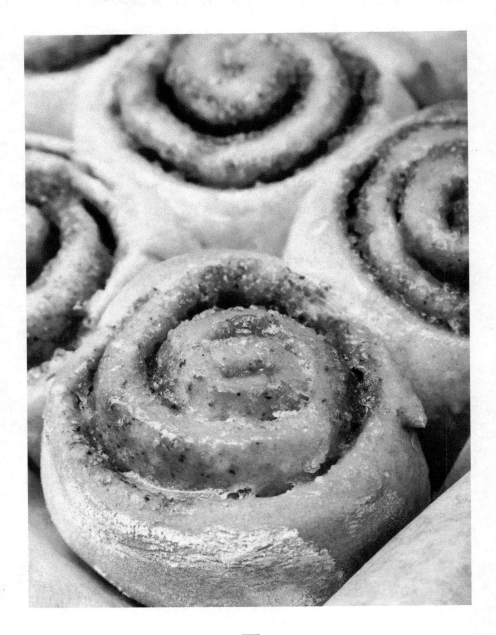

Ingredients:

3/4 cup milk - 4 tbsp. maple syrup - 1 ½ tbsp. active yeast - 1 tbsp. ground flaxseed - 1 tbsp coconut oil, melted - 1 cup flour - 1 ½ cup flour - 2 tsp cinnamon powder - ½ cup pecan nuts - 2 bananas, sliced - 4 Medjool dates, pitted - ¼ cup sugar

Instructions:

Warm the milk until it is tepid. Combine with the yeast and maple syrup, waiting 5 minutes to allow the yeast to activate. Put 3 tbsp of water and the flaxseed in a bowl and stir together. Let the flaxseed absorb the water for about 2 minutes. Pour the coconut oil into the bowl, then combine the flaxseed mixture with the yeast mixture. In a separate bowl, mix together one tbsp of the cinnamon powder and the white and flour. Add the yeast and flaxseed mixture and mix to create a dough. Dust a flat surface with flour and knead the dough with your hands for 10 minutes. Grease a large bowl and transfer the dough inside. Let sit in a warm, dark place for an hour so that the dough may rise. For the filling, mix the banana slices, dates, and pecans together before throwing in a tbsp of cinnamon powder. Set the Air Fryer to 390°F and allow it to warm. On your floured surface, flatten the dough with a rolling pin. Spoon the pecan mixture onto the dough and spread out evenly. Roll up the dough and slice. Transfer the slices to a dish small enough to fit in the fryer, set the dish inside, and cook for 30 minutes. Top with a thin layer of sugar.

Carrot Cake

6 Servings | 55 minutes

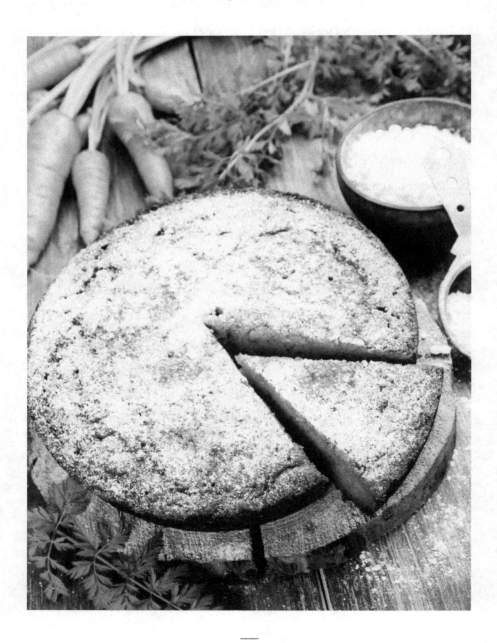

Ingredients:

Five ounces of flour - 3/4 teaspoon of baking powder - 1/2 teaspoon of baking soda - 1/2 teaspoon of ground cinnamon - Nutmeg 1/4 tsp., ground - 1/2 allspice teaspoon - 1 egg - Three yogurt spoons - 1/2 cups of sugar - 1/4 cup of pineapple juice - Four spoonfuls of sunflower oil - 1/3 cup of carrots, ground together - 1/3 cup of pecans, diced and toasted - 1/3 cup of crushed coconut flakes - Cooking spray

Instructions:

Mix the flour in a cup of baking soda and powder, salt and allspice, nutmeg, and cinnamon, then combine. Put the egg and yogurt, sugar, pineapple juice, oil, carrots in another dish.

Mix well and pecans and cocoa powder.

Merge the best mixtures and blend properly; pour into a spring pan that suits your fryer with cooking spray, which you grated with. Switch to your AirFryer and bake for 45 minutes at 320° F.

Let the cake cool off, then cut it down and serving it.

Chocolate Cake

4 Servings | 40 minutes

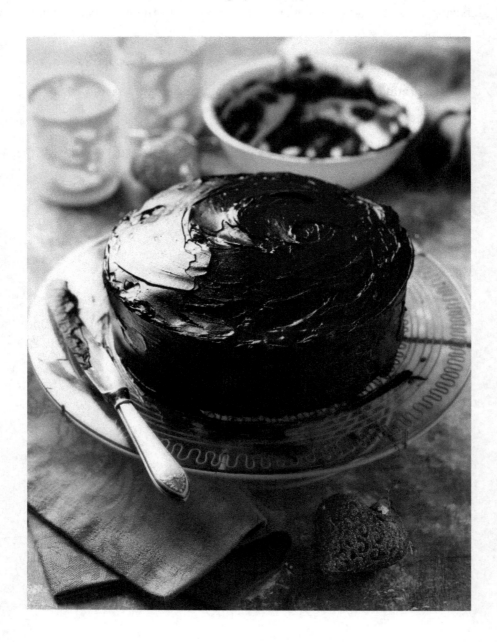

Ingredients:

½ cup of chopped dark chocolate, melted - 8 tablespoons of butter, melted - 5 tablespoons of sugar - ½ teaspoon of coffee - 1 teaspoon of baking powder - 2 eggs- 1 small lemon, juiced - 1/3 cup of flour - ¼ teaspoon of salt

Instructions:

Add the melted chocolate and the butter and lemon together and mix.
Put the egg, coffee, and sugar in a mixing bowl and whisk until creamy.

Add the chocolate-butter mixture and mix.
Add and stir the baking powder, flour, and salt. Mix the batter gently.

Heat your AirFryer to 356°F. Put the batter into a greased baking dish and place it in the fryer basket. Air fry for 10 minutes or until firm.

Peanut Butter Cookies

6 Servings | 15 minutes

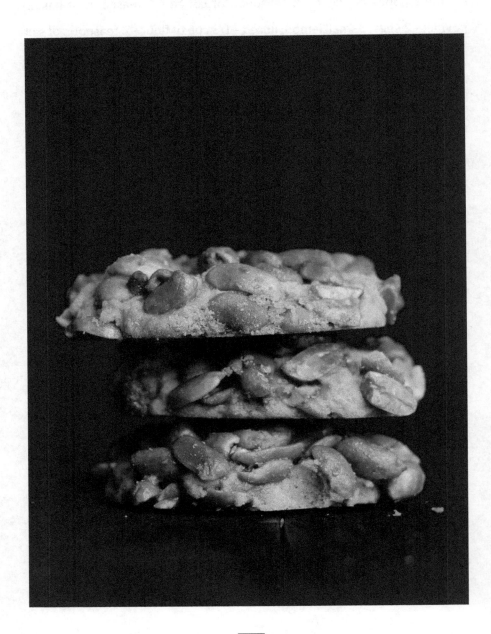

Ingredients:

1 cup of smooth peanut butter no-sugar-added - 1/3 cup of erythritol granular - 1 big egg - 1 teaspoon of vanilla extract

Instructions:

Combine all ingredients in a bowl until smooth. For 2 more minutes, begin stirring, and the mixture begins to thicken.

Roll out the mixture into eight balls and gently press to flatten out into 2 circular discs.

Cut parchment to match your air-freezer and Set it in a basket. Put the cookies on the basket Parchment—function as required in batches. Change the temperature and set the timer to 320° F for eight minutes. 5 Flip the 6-minute mark over the cookies. Serve and enjoy!

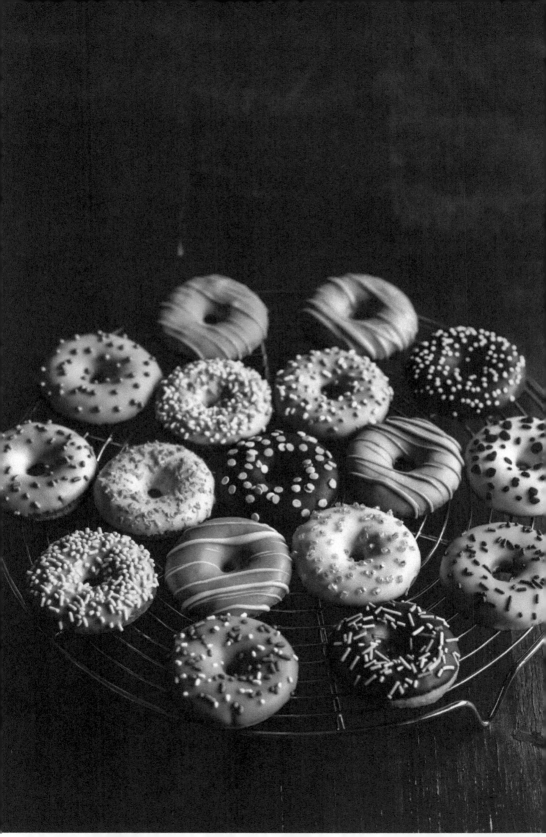

AMERICA'S RECIPES HUB

CPSIA information can be obtained
at www.ICGtesting.com
Printed in the USA
BVHW091739150521
607359BV00003B/436

9 781802 600117